MY POOL of BETHESDA

My Place of Healing and Transformation

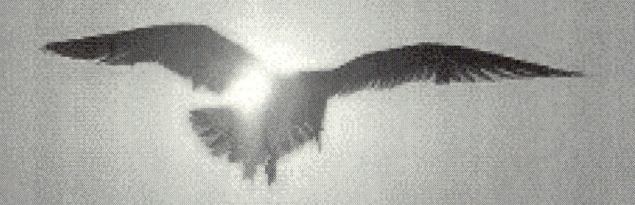

JENNIFER NSENKYIRE

MY POOL of BETHESDA

My Place of Healing and Transformation

Jennifer Nsenkyire

Copyright ©2018

Jennifer Nsenkyire

All Rights Reserved.

No portion of this publication may be reproduced, stored in any electronic system, or transmitted in any form or by any means (electronic, mechanical, photocopy, recording, or otherwise) without written permission from the publisher.

Brief quotations may be used in literary reviews.

ISBN: 978-0-359-03754-4

To DeeDee Mendez
I hope my story inspires you and gives you hope. It is great to know another patriot.

— [signature]
December 2019

This book is dedicated to:
Maame Yaa Gyamfuah my maternal grandmother.
Nana I thank God you lived to see me cured and no longer suffering with pain.
I thank you for your love and prayers.
My nieces and nephews, I pray this serves as a source of hope and encouragement to each one of you.

Acknowledgments

In spite of my medical trials and tribulations, my moments of hope inspired me to pen this Memoir. I did not get here overnight. It took the good Lord, dedication, family, friends and some very special people God placed in my life; and all of them deserve some very special thanks.

First and foremost, I would like to give thanks to God for His hand on my life. Without His mighty hand, I would not be where I am today. I made it this far in life because he had me in the palm of His hands. He has brought me through so much and I cannot imagine my life without Him. Without His guidance, this book would not have been written or published.

Secondly, I would like to thank my parents, Mr. and Mrs. E. O. Nsenkyire. I am grateful and blessed to have you as my parents. Your love and prayers through my many struggles is beyond words. God put me in your lives because He knew you would be the best support system for me. Your unconditional love and dedication is what has sustained me. There are not enough words in my vocabulary to express my love and appreciation. Also, to my siblings and their respective spouses: Mr. and Mrs., B.K. Asamoah, Mr. and Mrs. D. O. Nsenkyire and Clara Nsenkyire, your continued love, concern and support have been my source of strength. You reached out and touched me in areas when I was so far gone and could not be reached by most. You were able to touch and pull me through many challenges. I'd be lost without each and every one of you.

To Dr. and Mrs. Agyarko Bediako, your love, dedication and advice has been of great importance to me over the years. I thank you for being available to me when I needed you. I thank you for being my support system when my parents were far away. Your commitment is one only parent's like you can provide. My heart bursts with immense gratitude. To Grand Pa Alex Kwabena Owusu, your continued support is appreciated. To my extended family and friends who have impacted my life one way or the other and who are too many to list, my gratitude for your support is endless. To Mrs. Cecelia Beausoliel, Mrs. Naana Ampratwum, and Ms. Fran Boyle, I thank you for embracing me with consistent prayers, love and concern. Your availability and support through the many struggles I've experienced in life certainly helped strengthen my faith. God heard your prayers and collected the tears you shed in the palm of His hand and cleansed me with it.

Lastly, a special thanks to the late Harvey E. Johnson, Jr. and his family, whom until his departure from this world always ensured job security for me with his company. A special thanks to the doctors, nurses and staff of the Hematology Oncology Associates of Alexandria; and the doctors, nurses, specialists and staff of the National Institute and Health (NIH) and the National Heart Lung and Blood Institute (NHLBI) team, 3NE Medical Oncology/Haematology/Transplant Unit, 5NW General Medicine Unit, 5SE Inpatient Unit, Out Patient Clinic 7 Staff, and the Pain and

Palliative Care team. Minister Kiesha Patterson, a special thanks to you for your patience and guidance through this writing process. God definitely had a hand in connecting us. You started off as my writing coach, but we have built a friendship and a trust I believe will last a life time. I could not have achieved my goal of writing this book without you. You guided me through it all with great dedication and advice. It is the selflessness you exude, that shows your genuineness and commitment to others and your love for God.

Introduction

Like the man at the "Pool of Bethesda" in John 5 (New International Version, John 5:1-9), I had been at the pool wishing to be healed for years. I have often wondered why there was almost always something wrong with my health. I always seemed to have an issue going on medically. It seems as though I am a magnet for medical problems of various kinds. I cannot help but wonder why that is. Very often, I wonder what people think of me when they continuously hear of me encountering one medical problem after another. Some have commended me over the years on how strong they think I am to have endured all these challenges and still be able to put a smile on my face. I have been told I am brave to have gone through all that I have been through and still have a great attitude and approach to life. The interesting thing about all of this is that I never saw myself as being a strong person until recently. Rather, I saw myself as taking it one day at a time. On many occasions, it was a struggle for me to see the light in my world even when the sun was out. That is how dark my world had become.

For many years, I lived in pain and depression. I tried to make the best out of most days. I was discouraged, and beaten down by multiple illnesses; yet, I chose to make the best out of the hand I had been dealt. Though I did not want to fall into the "woe is me" pattern of life, I did. I fell in this pattern more often than I would like to admit. It was difficult trying not to stay in this space. I forced myself not to allow that feeling to take over. The love and support from family and friends I had around me sometimes helped me in dealing with the challenges. Another thing that kept me going during these trying periods was my faith. On most days, I felt so alone and frustrated at the hand I had been dealt. "When will it end?" and "When will it be enough?" were questions that constantly flooded my mind. The unhappiness and frustration I felt seeped into every area of my life. These feelings were projected directly towards me and my loved ones. I sought to end it all on many occasions. The anger and frustration towards my family was undeserving and unnecessary.

These last few years have been different. I have a lot to be thankful for. Regardless of the multiple medical challenges I have faced and still face, there have also been moments of hope to reflect upon. It is unfortunate it took these last few years for me to realize how blessed I am. I had so much to be thankful for and yet I was consumed with pain, frustration and anger. I had no time to focus on the positives. At the time, I just could not see anything positive happening in my life. I had a lot coming at me, one health challenge after another. There were so many ups and downs. I could not and did not see the light at the end of the tunnel. As I reflect back on my life, I realize I had a lot to be grateful for then and more so now. I will never allow myself to dwell in that "woe is me" space anymore. I consider myself blessed. In fact, I am extremely blessed.

My life now, is one I had only dreamt of. I never thought I would be in the space and place I am in today. Though I am still going through medical challenges, I do not and will not allow these negative feelings to creep in and cause me to forget how fortunate I am. I am enjoying the moment. I sometimes wonder if this is really me. It is amazing how incredible my life has been transformed. This thought crosses my mind often because the person I am now is completely different from the person I used to be. The person I used to be dwelt in the midst of unhealthy habits and behaviors. As a result, my life and vision was clouded with negativity on a daily basis. My life and world sucked! It was filled with a combination of:

- Depression
- Anger
- Irritability
- Chronic pain
- Frustration
- Worry
- Lack of faith
- Lack of self-control
- Lack of accountability
- Lack of self esteem
- Suicidal thoughts
- Addiction to prescription pain medicine

Bottom line, I was miserable. Oh Yes!!!! That was me THEN. The key word is **THEN**. By the Grace of God things have changed. God has changed my identity. Those things that used to be a part of me are no longer so. By God's grace I am no longer who I used to be. I have made a complete 360 degree turn in life. This transformation has altered my whole outlook on life.

Today, my mentality, attitude, and view of myself are positive. I am stronger than I have ever been in mind, body and soul. I am confident; I am happier and no longer depressed. I am accountable for my actions, now trustworthy and do encompass a mind with strong self-control. The negative things listed above are no longer a representation of who I am today. This list is now foreign to me. It is foreign because I like my current life better. In hindsight, I now realize how debilitating a negative mindset can affect one's life. I cannot fathom having lived in such misery for so long. My "world" and vision were clouded.

What caused the transformation? I hope there is a peak in your interest? Continue reading to find out what that significant change was that impacted my life. God has done a lot for me. In fact, He has done great things for me. I am even amazed at what He has done and continue to do in my life. People are in awe when they see me and hear my story. My dear friend, I do know and have experienced first-hand that God is the same yesterday, today and forever. God does not and will not change. When I decided to place my complete trust in Him and surrender, He delivered me. After thirty-eight and half years, He answered my most intimate prayer. God answered my prayer and granted me the healing I had longed for. The healing I had asked for and longed for was finally granted when I finally made a conscious effort to trust and believe in God. Yes, He did it for me and will do it for you. My dear friend, here is my story and I hope and pray it impacts your life profoundly.

Chapter 1

It all started in 1973, on a beautiful Wednesday morning in Cape Coast, Ghana. Rose Nsenkyire was pregnant and ready to have the little bundle of joy she had been carrying in her belly for the past nine months. She had been in labor for a few hours prior to arriving at the Cape Coast Central Hospital to have her child delivered. Both Rose and Edward Nsenkyire, her husband, were eager in anticipation of the newest addition to their family. At the time, there were no ultra sounds, sonograms, or tests that could determine the sex and or health of the baby. Yet, the proud parents were content in that. They trusted the God who had given them two healthy children, a daughter and a son, would once again give them a healthy and beautiful child; and frankly, that was all that mattered to them. Rose went to the Cape Coast hospital in the Central Region of Ghana ready to bear this precious and active baby she had been carrying in her extended belly.

Cape Coast Central Hospital is located in the Central Region of Ghana. Ghana's Central Region is one of the ten administrative regions in the country. It is bordered by the Ashanti and Eastern regions to the north, the Western region to the west, the Greater Accra region to the east, and to the south by the Gulf of Guinea. The Central Region is renowned for its many elite higher educational institutions such as the Mfantsipim School, Wesley Girls High School, Adisadel College, and the St. Augustine's College. Cape Coast occupies an area of about 9,800 square kilometers, making it the third smallest region compared to the Greater Accra and the Upper East Regions of Ghana. The region was also one of the first area in the country to make contact with the Europeans who settled here and built trading lodges along the coast. Cape Coast was also the capital of the Gold Coast until 1877, when the capital was moved to Accra. It was in the castle of Cape Coast that the historic Bond of 1844 was signed between the British and the Fante Confederation.

Rose, accompanied by her husband and her mother, the late Maame Yaa Gyamfuah, checked into the maternity ward that early Wednesday morning. The drive to and check in at the hospital had been easy. They were all hopeful the birth of the child would be just as easy. After all, the pregnancy had been an easy one with no complications whatsoever. An easy birth would mean she would get to go home after a day or two. After a few more hours of being in labor she was ready to have her baby. The parents had agreed this would be their last child. They both wanted to focus on achieving other goals they had set for themselves both individually and as a family. Maame Yaa, as she was affectionately called, was just as elated about welcoming another grand-child. After all, Rose was her eldest daughter and she had certainly made Maame Yaa proud in more ways than she could imagine.

Rose was a great mother; she was also an outstanding third grade teacher climbing up the professional ladder steadily. As the oldest daughter, she had done almost everything right in her mother's eyes. Maame Yaa supported her daughter in all her endeavors both educationally and professionally. Her eldest daughter had exceeded her expectations by managing to juggle both motherhood and a career in teaching without missing a beat. Rose hardly called on her mother for advice or support in caring for her children or taking care of her household. Though she had a lot to juggle, with Edward travelling quite often for work all over the world and having guests in her home either for just a meal or to visit for a period of time, she took on these responsibilities with such grace, strength and determination.

At the time Edward was serving as the Conservator of Forests in the Forestry Department in Cape Coast. The family had been transferred from the Ashanti Region to the Central Region a few years prior. Their time in Cape Coast had been exciting thus far. They had made a ton of friends since their arrival there and had taken the opportunity to familiarize themselves with the town. In fact, Rose had been raised partly in Elmina, a fishing town not far from Cape Coast, by her father Albert Asante.

Chapter 2

The strong and determined mother was excited to have her third child and could not wait to see her baby's face, touch it and love it. After a few strong and deliberate pushes, wringing in pain and a little encouragement from the nurses in her care, Rose finally gave birth at approximately 7 am on the 7th day of February, 1973. She pushed into this world a beautiful and vivacious baby girl. The baby was delivered with a full head of hair and beautiful long "slits" for an eye. These long openings would widen just enough a couple of hours later to reveal the beautiful brown eyes hiding behind them. Those almond shaped eyes would enlarge just a little bit later to reveal more of those big brown eyes. She cried out loudly exercising her little lungs and for attention. Those almond shaped eyes would open to see the faces of a few of the doctors and nurses that had assisted in this momentous occasion, looking down and smiling at her.

Little did anyone know those eyes would shed many tears as a result of pain it would sustain over the years. Those eyes did not only shed tears of hunger or for her mother's attention as is typical of most children but it would also shed tears of pain, hurt, heartache, and frustration at the hand it had been dealt. Many tears poured out of those beautiful eyes for many years carrying an incredible story, one that will amaze many. It carried a story worth sharing with others and one that would make people realize and understand that no matter what challenges one faces in life, there are moments of hope hidden along the way. Over the years, those eyes would often plead, urge, and wonder when this pain would end, yet, relief seemed elusive. The relief those eyes sought on many occasions would be so evasive. Those eyes would be windows to a soul, a heart that has endured many struggles, many trials and yet continues to smile and show strength and courage within.

It was a joy for the parents and everyone including extended family members and friends that day. It had been an easy birth compared to other births at the Cape Coast Central Hospital. In fact, everything about this pregnancy and birth had been easy. After a couple of days in the hospital, mother and child were discharged to go home. Pamela and Dennis, the older siblings, were excited to have their baby sister home. They had been looking forward to this day for months, and to see it come to fruition gave them an excitement they could hardly contain. They were both on their best behavior and ready to lend a helping hand whenever Mommy needed it. They were extremely excited and gushed over their baby sister and argued over whose turn it was to help Mommy with the baby. They could hardly wait to come home from school to play with her. They shared the news with their friends and anyone who would listen to them at school.

Eight days after the birth, the precious baby was named Jennifer Adwoa Abrafi Nsenkyire. And that baby girl was me. I was named during an out-dooring ceremony which is referred to as the abadinto, by the Ashanti tribe of Ghana. The out-dooring ceremony is a custom practiced my many of the tribes in Ghana. This ceremony is a major celebration and a sign of welcoming the child not only into the family but also into society and the world. Traditionally the naming ceremony begins early in the morning. It is the father of the new born who is tasked with the responsibility of giving a name to the child. As a norm, the extended family members and friends meet in the early morning to support the parents in undertaking this important task. The father makes the decision on the name and presents the child to the family notifying them of the names the child is to be called. After the father presents the child and the name to the family, an elder in the family dips the tip of his finger into water and touches the child's tongue. The elder then dips his hand into alcohol and touches the child's tongue a second time. The significance of this practice is for the child to be able to differentiate right from wrong and to know truth from lies and live by those guidelines.

As part of the custom, the out-dooring ceremony was followed with a celebration which included food, drinks, music and dancing; as well as, the company of many friends and family members some of whom traveled miles to join in on this festive occasion.

Chapter 3

Not long after my birth, my Dad was transferred from Cape Coast to the headquarters of the Forestry Department in Accra. Accra is the political and economic capital of Ghana. Between the years of 1500 and 1578, a fortress operated by the Portuguese stood at the site of modern Accra. This fort provided the Europeans with an outlet for trade, particularly in slaves, with the Ga people. In 1642, the Dutch expelled the Portuguese from the Gold Coast and established a new trading post at Accra. In the early 1660s, the Company of Royal Adventurers of England Trading to Africa would later establish a series of posts in the region igniting a war between the English and the Dutch over the Gold Coast trade domination. After the treaty of Breda in 1672, the victorious English formed their trading post in Accra which was eventually expanded into a fortress. In 1877, the colonial capital was moved from the traditional center of British power at Cape Coast to Accra. Throughout the colonial era, Accra preserved its prominence as the center for trade. Even after the construction of a deep water port at Takoradi town in the Western Region in 1928, Accra's surf port remained economically and politically significant in more ways than one. During the Second World War, Accra became an important link in the Allied transportation network between the European and East Asian regions of the conflict. After Ghana became the first sub-Saharan African colony to gain independence in 1957, the first

Prime Minister Kwame Nkrumah assured the local population that Accra would remain the capital, which it did.

Although this transfer for my Dad and the family was expected, it had come rather quickly considering we had just moved to Cape Coast less than four years earlier. However, as duty called, off we packed and left this town they were still exploring. The move to Accra was viewed as one that would be beneficial to everyone in the family. Accra offered a great deal more than what Cape Coast had to offer. Being that, Accra is the capital city of Ghana, it offered a close proximity and accessibility to governmental agencies and access to more modern medical facilities. Accra offered more and better equipped schools that would open up opportunities for my mother as a teacher and for us, the children. It also offered exposure to new and exciting activities for the family as a whole to engage in. In short the move to this new place would be beneficial to all.

The Nsenkyire's arrival in Accra was met with a warm welcome by the team at the Forestry Department of Ghana. The family was welcomed with a three bedroom bungalow and a car. Not only did Pam and Dennis love their new home but they also loved the huge compound that came with it and could not wait to explore it. Edward's hard work and dedication had paid off. This move was the result of a promotion for Edward. The promotion was for him to become the Headquarters Assistant of the Forestry

Department. Though this move was exciting, he also knew it came with it a lot more travel and responsibilities. But, Edward was in for the challenge. He never shied away from hard work; a quality he and Rose tried to instill in us. While Edward adjusted to his new role, Rose was busy finding new schools for Pam and Dennis to attend while nursing her new born. Eventually, Rose also secured a teaching position at the Kotobabi Presbyterian Primary School where she taught until her voluntary retirement in the late 1980s.

Chapter 4

Like most babies I was growing up beautifully and strong. I would experience the occasional cold, cough or malaria every now and then and had no medical issues out of the ordinary. For those of you who do not know what Malaria is, it can be life-threatening. It is typically transmitted through the bite of an infected Anopheles mosquito. Infected mosquitoes carry the Plasmodium parasite. When this mosquito bites you, the parasite is released into your bloodstream. Once the parasites are inside your body, they travel to the liver, where they mature. After several days, the mature parasites enter the bloodstream and begin to infect the red blood cells. Within 48 to 72 hours, the parasites inside the red blood cells multiply, causing the infected cells to burst open. The parasites continue to infect the red blood cells, resulting in symptoms that occur in cycles that last two to three days at a time. Malaria is typically found in tropical and subtropical climates where the parasites can live.

Very often I would get over these illnesses just as easily and as quickly as most children would. However, when I was about a year and a half old, I started experiencing pain and swelling in my arms or legs quite frequently. My parents began to notice quite often that an arm or a leg would swell up and hurt without any cause or aggravation. The swelling would linger on for a few days and subside with the application of mild medication and/or a heating pad. This went on for a few years and eventually, my parents decided to seek medical attention at the Korle-Bu Teaching Hospital, which was and still is a major health facility in Accra, Ghana.

Established on October 9, 1923, the Korle Bu Teaching Hospital has grown from an initial 200 to 2,000 bed capacity. This facility is currently the third largest hospital in Africa and the leading national referral center in Ghana. Korle Bu, which means the valley of the Korle lagoon, was established as a General Hospital to address the general health concerns of the indigenous people under Sir Gordon Guggisberg's administration. Sir Gordon Guggisberg was the then Governor of the Gold Coast. Population growth and the proven worth of hospital-based treatment resulted in an increase in hospital attendance at Korle Bu. By 1953, demand for the Hospital's services had increased so greatly; as a result, the government was compelled to expand it and to increase the hospital's bed capacity. This expansion brought about the construction of new structures, such as the Maternity, Medical, Surgical and Children's Health Blocks.

Korle Bu gained teaching hospital status in 1962, when the University of Ghana Medical School (UGMS) was established for the training of medical doctors. The UGMS and five other schools are now included under the College of Health Sciences to train various health professionals. At the moment, the Hospital has 2,000 beds as mentioned earlier and 17 clinical and diagnostic departments. It has an average daily attendance of 1,500 patients and an estimated 250 patient admissions. Clinical and diagnostic departments of the Hospital include Medicine, Child Health, Obstetrics and Gynecology, Pathology, Laboratories, Radiology, Anesthesia, Surgery, Polyclinic, Accident Centre and the Surgical/Medical Emergency as well as Pharmacy.

It was at the Korle Bu Teaching Hospital that my parents met the late Dr. Joseph Tawiah Bonney Quaye. At this facility, my parents would finally get the answers they needed. Dr. Quaye was the kind of doctor who not only took care of the patient, but also ensured the caregivers were well educated enough about a diagnosis. He was gentle, patient, compassionate, confident and knowledgeable, yet humble. Being a pediatrician and having a love for children, Dr. Quaye was in a field he was passionate about. After observing me over a number of visits and initiating a number of medical tests, Dr. Quaye finally concluded I had Sickle Cell Disease (SCD) just as he had suspected initially. As people used to refer to patients with SCD back then, I was a "sickler". He went into detail by explaining to my parents what SCD meant and how I had acquired it. This revelation was a total surprise to them. It was a surprise because they did not know a whole lot about it and how it is passed on to an offspring. Further tests confirmed both of my parents were carriers of the disease. This implied that both parents had the AS genotype or trait. In my case, since both parents had the Sickle Cell trait, it meant they both carried an S gene and thus the two S genes were passed on to me and having two S genes (SS) caused me to have the form of SCD called Sickle Cell Anemia.

Chapter 5

For those of you who are not familiar with the disease, SCD is a group of inherited red blood cells with abnormal hemoglobin called hemoglobin S or sickle hemoglobin (a protein in red blood cells that carries oxygen throughout the body). People who have SCD inherit two abnormal hemoglobin genes, one from each parent. There are many forms of SCD. When a person has two hemoglobin S genes, that is, Hemoglobin SS, the disease is called Sickle Cell Anemia. This is the most common and often most severe kind of SCD. Hemoglobin SC disease and hemoglobin Sβ thalassemia (thal-uh-SEE-me-uh) are two other common forms of SCD. Cells in tissues need a steady supply of oxygen to work well. Normally, hemoglobin in red blood cells takes up oxygen in the lungs and carries it to all the tissues of the body. Red blood cells that contain normal hemoglobin are disc shaped. This shape allows the cells to be flexible enabling it to move through large and small blood vessels to deliver oxygen. The Sickle hemoglobin is abnormal hemoglobin which can form stiff rods within the red cell, changing it into a crescent, or sickle shape. Sickle-shaped cells are not flexible and can stick to vessel walls, causing a blockage that slows or stops the flow of blood. When this occurs, oxygen cannot reach nearby tissues. It is not contagious. In other words, a person cannot catch it, like a cold or infection, from someone else.

Though this diagnosis was not what my parents were expecting, they embraced the facts of the diagnosis and asked questions. It was a wakeup call and it also served as an opportunity for them to educate themselves and help educate others. The diagnosis brought to light important discussions my family needed to have about the disease. For my family, it brought to light the need for awareness and education. I am fortunate to have been born to parents who were well educated and open to embracing the diagnosis, its implications and use of modern medicine. Even to this day in the twenty first century, there continues to be a lack of awareness, acceptance and education in many West African countries. Quite often, instead of families accepting a diagnosis, they tend to believe it is either a curse on the family or a curse on the individual with the diagnosis. Thus, instead of seeking modern medical care, the family turns to traditional or local doctors for care. This can be detrimental to the patient.

Although educated and fairly widely traveled at the time, my parents did not know extensively about this disease like most Ghanaians. They were also not prepared for what was to come. I thank God they had found their way to the Korle-Bu Teaching Hospital and into the hands and care of Dr. Quaye. With the late Dr. Quaye's knowledge, assistance and direction, my parents were educated on what to expect and how to handle pain crises. Pain crisis became my norm or should I say our norm as a family. My parents did everything they possibly could to help me deal with the pain. Whether it was medication or food they believed could help alleviate the intensity and frequency of the pain crises, my parents gladly sought it out. They were committed to assisting me deal with this disease as best as they could.

Chapter 6

Over the years, I went through numerous and frequent pain crises. With most of these crises, I was hospitalized for days, if not months. The pain crisis could be triggered by different things. Some were a result of dehydration, anemia and/or malaria. I endured many prolonged hospital stays for this reason. Receiving blood transfusions and intravenous fluids became quite frequent and continued on even through my adult life. Those big brown eyes shed tears on many nights for this pain to end.

Experiencing these bouts of pain which often resulted in subsequent visit to hospitals like the Nyaho Clinic or the Korle-Bu hospital often caused an interruption in my life. It was interrupting my life in the sense that I was missing out on being a regular normal child. I was missing out on life period. While my siblings and neighborhood kids enjoyed their childhood, I was either in the hospital or at home nursing my pain. I felt left out and alone while my siblings engaged in activities regular kids participated in. I felt left out not because my siblings purposefully left me out. I felt left out because of the toll these bouts of pain crisis took on me. While my mates were at school learning; building mental and social skills; building friendships, I was on admission at the hospital taking classes from the hospital appointed teacher. While they hopped and ran outside in the sun yelling and screaming at each other, I was alone in my hospital bed in excruciating pain.

When I was not in pain, I was like any other child who got in trouble every now and then from mischief. Like most children my age, I had chores, homework and friends to think about. I loved playing outside; and enjoyed playing house with my siblings and friends from the neighborhood. If I did something wrong, be it lying or eating something I was not supposed to eat, my parents did not spare me. I was treated like my siblings where certain actions and behaviors resulted in consequences such as time out. And for that I remain grateful to my parents for not treating me any different. I am happy I was treated the same way regardless of how often or how severely SCD affected me. I am appreciative of the fact that they gave me a childhood close to normal as they possibly could. I was not sheltered or treated in any special way.

Chapter 7

Approximately three years after my birth, my parents had another child, a daughter whom they would name Clara. Not long after the birth of this child, my parents had her tested for SCD. As fate would have it, the tests revealed she also carried the disease. Clara was diagnosed as having the two SS genes like I did. By this time my two older siblings had been tested and both Pamela and Dennis turned out to be just carriers. This meant they both had the trait and not the disease. Just like it had been explained to us, if both parents have the Sickle Cell trait there is a likelihood some of their children will have the trait and the others will have the disease. This explains why Pamela and Dennis had the trait while Clara and I have the disease.

God's amazing love and grace worked it out whereby the manifestation of the disease in my younger sibling's life was not as severe as it was in mine. Her condition did not impact her as gravely, in that she was able to engage in and participate in various strenuous activities I was unable to engage in. Her education and or attendance at school were hardly impacted by this disease. In fact, she very rarely fell ill. It was to a point where we doubted she had been correctly diagnosed. When Clara was about ten years of age, my parents had her retested, and of course, the results came back the same as before, which was no surprise. It was like night and day when you compared my condition to hers. Our cases were completely different in that if you compared how often and how severe I got sick to that of hers, it was mind boggling. It may have been mind boggling to us, but like in the case of any other disease, its manifestation in each individual is different. Although, I think it was God's way of giving this family, these parents, and siblings a break. I strongly believe it was His way of saying one severe case is enough for this family. I could not imagine what our lives would have been like, had my younger sister's diagnosis been any other way. I think about this often and I know God works in mysterious ways indeed that we as human beings will never understand.

On the rare occasions when Clara and I were in severe pain crises and ended up on admission, the nurses and doctors would arrange for us to share a room. Knowing this, Clara would sometimes fake a pain crisis, just so she could be with me at the hospital. As a young child she could not comprehend why her sister was always in some sort of pain. She could not fathom why her sister was always in and out of the hospital. Even when I was home, there were a lot of activities I was unable to engage in. Simple and fun activities like swimming would send me into a major crisis. Clara would often ask my parents questions as to why I was always sick and unable to engage in certain activities like most kids. My parents patiently educated her the best way a child could understand. She just could not understand why I was away from home and get to stay away from school for weeks on end. It was difficult for her to watch me in pain on many occasions. And sometimes, she wished there was something she could do to take away some of the pain her sweet sister was facing.

Chapter 8

Many nights I woke up from sleep in pain. These bouts of pain would often start off in the form of a dream. In the dream, I would experience pain in my chest, arms, legs and or lower back just like a real pain crisis. In the dream I would moan, toss and turn from the intense pain. I would awaken suddenly from this dream only to realize the intense pain and discomfort were not a dream after all. It would always turn out to be a reality. It would always turn out to be a reality I did not want to face. Once I woke up with the pain crisis well underway, I would take a regimen of pain medication, coupled with plenty of fluids to help the pain subside. It is believed the fluids assist in the circulation and the flow of the sickle shaped cells through the veins. This helps loosen the cells which are stuck together and unable to flow freely. Sometimes the cocktail of medications would help relieve the pain and I would be able to go back to sleep. On many other occasions, even with fluids and pain medicine, the crisis would linger on for hours and sometimes days.

On many occasions, I would have to be taken to the hospital for stronger pain medication and intravenous fluids. Sometimes I would get admitted for observation over a period of time in instances where I was dehydrated or had some sort of on-going infection. The length of stay varied depending on what the underlying issue was. The period of stay could very well be over a number of days, weeks or even months. I would often receive numerous blood transfusions, intravenous fluids and a variety of medications, including antibiotics of various kinds. That was my life. I was anemic almost always due to this disease. Although my parents did their best in ensuring I consumed overall a healthy diet, I could not seem to make enough red blood cells and stayed anemic.

My parents were always in search of the next healthy protein filled juice, meal or snack for my siblings and I. In our home, there was almost always a new meal idea introduced as long as it was believed to be beneficial in helping us, especially Clara and I to boost our protein levels. My Mom would ensure eggs were part of our daily breakfast for instance. Although Pam and Dennis seemed to enjoy their breakfast with no qualms, Clara and I did not enjoy eating eggs no matter the manner in which it was prepared. We just disliked eating eggs especially the yolk. We threw the yolk under our dining table each and every time it was served to us and pretend we had eaten it. In our minds, getting rid of it this way was the smartest idea because one side of our dining table sat against a wall. Our parents never looked underneath or behind that dining table, so we thought. Needless to say my Mom found multiple egg yolks underneath the dining table one day and was very upset with Clara and I. My parent's quest to ensure we had a nutrient filled diet never stopped. They tried everything from liver, yoghurt, cheese, and beverages of various kinds.

I was not allowed to engage in any strenuous activities such as sports and Physical Education (PE). I wanted to join my peers in these activities but was forbidden to engage in them and also because anytime I did, I would go into crisis. At school some of my teachers treated me as though I was fragile. On one occasion, I was told by a teacher not to run because I could break a bone. I despised being treated in this manner and often wished people around me would not view me as sick or helpless. I despised being called a "sickler". One other thing I detested was when people viewed me with pity. Pity was not what I needed. Rather, I needed empathy, encouragement and support. The look of pity was and is depressing to me. It made me feel sorry for myself; thus, influencing me to focus more on the disease and how it prevented me from living a normal life. I believe the lack of knowledge about the disease was also why people reacted to or treated me the way they did when they find out I have SCD. For those who were empathetic and always provided support and/or joined my family and in prayer, I will forever be grateful.

Often times I felt isolated, especially at school and among friends. I would watch them engage in activities I wished I could participate in. My only consolation was that, I was never treated differently by my family. My parents treated me just like they would treat my siblings. I had chores and responsibilities in the home. I was scolded and grounded when I was disobedient or disrespectful.

The only times I was treated differently was when I was having a pain crisis. In fact, to this day, my parents value the one important advice the late Dr. Quaye gave them. He always reminded them not to treat me any differently from my siblings. This advice was very helpful because it allowed me to shed off the feeling of isolation when I walked through the doors of our home. I also felt guilty for taking up much of my parent's time and attention from my siblings. This guilt weighed heavily on me as a child and I often wished there was something I could do to change that.

Chapter 9

At nine years old, I developed complications from Osteomyelitis, a rare but serious bone infection that affected my limbs. With this infection, bones can become infected in a number of ways. Infection in one part of the body may spread through the bloodstream into the bone, or an open fracture or surgery may expose the bone to infection. This condition affects children and adults in various ways. Certain conditions and behaviors that weaken ones immune system can increase the risk for Osteomyelitis.

I do not have a clear recollection of exactly how it all started. However, what I do recall was that it started off with swelling and pain in my left leg. In my case, the infection eventually affected all four limbs. Due to the severity of the infection, and my inability to use my limbs, I was admitted at Korle-Bu Hospital. While on admission, all four limbs were placed in a cast for a period of time. The purposes of the casts were to help the bones to heal. The casts were half casts and wrapped with bandages. The bandages were unwrapped occasionally for the doctors to examine the bone. As a result of the infection I developed a wound around the chin of my left leg. The nurses would attend to the wound unpacking gauze soaked in blood and repacking fresh new gauze into it. The wound was so severe that eventually, I underwent surgery to have the puss drained from it. I would cry out in excruciating pain whenever the wound was attended to. This pain was worse than any pain I had ever experienced. I was essentially bed-ridden and at the mercy of my doctors and nurses. My parents visited daily while my mom and grandmother took turns spending the nights with me.

The hospital ward, in which I was an inpatient, had about three or four other children occupying a room. Over time we formed a friendship. We each were in the hospital for different reasons and struggled through them together. We developed a relationship, a bond that not only held us together but also helped pull us through the difficult times we each faced. Our parents cultivated friendships as well. They relied on, supported and encouraged each other. They served as a support system for all of the children. My siblings; friends from church, school and the neighborhood would visit occasionally to cheer me up. I would receive encouraging cards and Bible verses from family and friends. These cards and bible verses adorned my wall and served as a reminder of the love and support that surrounded me. These served as a reminder of the prayers that were coming my way. The love shown towards me was very encouraging. I relied on the scriptures as a source of encouragement always drawing spiritual strength from the messages that reminded me God was on my side. I consistently trusted in Him and prayed for healing.

Most nights, I would read through my cards and scriptures. During a period in time when I needed the most encouragement, I received a scripture from my dear brother who like the other siblings and friends would send me scriptures periodically. On this occasion, the scripture that caught my attention and encouraged me the most was one that Dennis had written in one of his cards to me. It was as if he knew my secret. It was as if Dennis knew of my fear of not being able to ever walk again. It was as if he knew exactly what I was feeling and knew these words would help alleviate my fear. In this card, Dennis quoted: *Then Peter said, "Silver or gold I do not have, but what I do have I give you. In the name of Jesus Christ of Nazareth, walk." (New International Version, Acts 3:6).* This scripture meant so much to me and gave me the courage to know that I would be able to walk again.

In my sleep one night, after reading this scripture, I had a dream I will never forget. This dream was revealing and impactful on my life. In the dream I was asleep in my hospital bed when I felt someone come into my room and touch me. This touch was soft and gentle, like that of a feather. Even though this touch was like the brush of a feather, it felt as though it was one intended to wake me up. It was intended to get me out of my sleep. The touch awakened me and as I opened my eyes, I saw a man standing at the foot of my bed. The man looked like Jesus. He had long hair and the same facial features as the picture of Jesus in the Bible stories I had read.

In the dream, the man looked at me with a gentle smile and said, "Jennifer, can you walk?" It was as if I knew this man from before. I was not in the least scared and calmly answered "yes". As he stood with a gentle smile on his face, he extended his arm and said "Jennifer get up and walk." In the dream I slowly got up out of the bed, stood up and began to walk towards him. At this point in the dream I did not see the casts. Somehow somewhere the casts and bandages had fallen off my arms and legs. I no longer saw the limitations. I no longer saw the hindrances. I no longer felt any fear. They had fallen off me. In the dream I was able to walk normally as if I had never been in the casts for the extended period of time. I walked as if I had been using my legs every day. After taking a few steps towards Him, I suddenly became aware of my surroundings, realizing it had all been a dream. Although it was all a dream, I was extremely excited to share this with my mother the following morning. For me, this dream was an indication of things to come. This dream to me meant I would be able to walk again and I was excited to share this. Even at that young age, I felt God would do great things in my life. Even at that young age of nine, I knew the significance of the dream and believed in it so strongly.

I had a big smile on my face, when my mother walked through the doors to my hospital room and came towards my bed that morning. I started rumbling on about the dream even before she got to my bed. She requested that I slow down as she could not understand or follow a word I was saying as a result of my rumbling. As she patiently listened to my dream, I saw a smile form on her face. She was happy to hear the dream and especially how it all ended. Mom started to get me ready for the day as she needed to head back to the house to attend to other matters. She encouraged me to share my story with the doctors and the medical team when they came through for their daily rounds. She encouraged me not to entertain any fear moving forward. Even though I wished she would stay and help me share my story with the doctors, I unwillingly bid her good bye as she walked out the door.

Chapter 10

A few hours after my mother left, the team of doctors caring for me arrived for their morning rounds. As they walked up to my bed, the lead doctor, who was also the Orthopedic Surgeon who had orchestrated this whole recovery process, stood in the exact spot the man in my dream had stood the night before in my dream. It felt like de ja vu. After a couple of minutes of discussions among themselves, the surgeon asked me the same question I had been asked in the dream. He asked, "Jennifer can you walk?" I immediately responded with a resounding "Yes!" The only response I had to give was going to be a yes of course.

How could I respond any other way? After the experience I had in the dream, after the feeling of confidence and strength I had felt in my legs, there were no limitations and my answer to the team of doctors was going to be a yes. He proceeded to ask the nurse to remove the bandages and casts. The nurse slowly and carefully removed the bandages as ordered. In my mind this nurse was taking way too long to get these casts off. I was ready and excited about this opportunity! Once they were removed, the doctor examined all four limbs and the wound. After a few discussions among the team, I was asked to walk. He extended his hand out to me just like it had happened in the dream. This was my moment of truth. I slowly got off the bed, while holding on tightly to his extended arm, I stood up. Initially, I felt my legs were shaky or should I say unstable. But I was determined to rise to this occasion. I was determined not to be discouraged. I began taking steps towards the doctor. After a few steps, the doctor asked my nurse to assist me in walking further to strengthen my legs as he let go of my hand. Although I was terrified, I did not reveal this feeling in any manner to the doctors, nurses and those around me. In my mind, it was a dream come true to be able to walk and I was not going to allow fear to stop me in my tracks.

My legs felt wobbly in the beginning but I was determined to keep going. The doctors, nurses and everyone in the room who knew me and knew what I had been through was not only amazed, but happy to see me out of the bed I had been confined to for months. I could not and would not sit that day as shaky as my steps were. My nurse walked with me to all three floors of the children's block that morning. It did not matter to me how quivery my steps were, I was happy to be taking these steps to freedom. The nurse attending to my care encouraged me and with each step, my legs felt stronger.

Later that afternoon, my Mom returned to the hospital to check on me again. As she approached my bed, she realized I was not there. Someone finally shared the news with her. She was thrilled to hear that I was up and walking, but at the same time, she was not surprised by this news at all. She was filled with joy and so was everyone else who heard the news that day, both family and friends. I continued to stay at the hospital for a few more days for further observation and physical therapy. After being released from the hospital, I continued in physical therapy for a few more months. After months of physical therapy, my limbs gained strength and stability again. Even after all those months of therapy, I was never able to straighten my right arm fully. To this day it is slightly bent at the elbow and is always a reminder of what I went through during this period of my life. The wound on my leg eventually healed and also left a huge scar from the trauma that had ensued in that leg.

This experience was one of many traumatic hurdles I've had to face over the years. Even after this experience, I continually struggled with varying aspects of SCD. I missed school for weeks quite often. Yet each time I worked hard to catch up with my class mates. Each time I would claw my way back to the top with my mates. My parents had instilled in me the importance of hard work, commitment and dedication. In my struggles and challenges of living with Sickle Cell Anemia, I appreciated the importance of working even harder. Though it was a struggle trying to catch up on school work, I never gave up. I kept trying each and every time I was left behind. Through these struggles, my faith would wane. I found myself discouraged quite often.

My faith was tested on many occasions with the frequent hospital visits. Just when I thought I was clear of one problem, another developed. I struggled to be strong in faith. How could I remain grounded in faith when it was difficult to comprehend the hand I had been dealt. How could I remain grounded in faith, when I knew Sickle Cell disease had no cure. How could I remain grounded in faith, when it was my understanding that this was going to be how I would have to live my life and for as long as I had breath in me. I must admit there were days when the feeling of "woe is me" took over my thoughts. Yes, it was so strong sometimes I could not see any light at the end of the tunnel. What light? How could there be any light at the end of this tunnel? There were days I wished it would all end. There were days I wished the pain would end. There were times when I felt I was a burden on my family, although that was far from the truth. But that is what pain, despair, helplessness and anger can do to anyone. I began to imagine things that did not really exist. I also took everything so personally.

Chapter 11

I went through my teenage years the same way I did as a young child. There were many hospital stays during which family and friends would visit with me. I cherished visits from my friends the most. It was an opportunity for them to get me caught up on what I had missed at school or on news from the neighborhood. It was my opportunity to feel connected to my peers. We would talk for hours on end, and would joke and tease each other. These were also moments that helped me take my mind off the pain and other medical challenges I endured. When in pain, I could often see the frustration in the eyes of family and friends as they stood helpless and looked on. They were helpless because there was nothing they could do to alleviate this awful pain. My Grandmother would occasionally spend the night at the hospital with me. She would bring my favorite candy from Kumasi to cheer me up. When the pain crisis was intense, nothing could help take my mind off it. Not even my favorite candy or meal. I always looked forward to being discharged from the hospital; going home to my own bed and joining my friends back at school. Just when I would feel like things were back to normal, I would get sick again and go through another repetition of this cycle.

Although this was unusual for most kids and their families, these hospital visits became the norm for me and my family. As much as I was pampered and cared for by my loved ones during these times, I did not enjoy going through these painful moments and the frequency with which it occurred. Pain crisis became part of my identity. If I ever missed an event or social gathering, everyone automatically assumed I was in crisis and probably on admission again. I was known as someone who was always ill, hence the name "sickler". Of course there were others who sometimes felt I was faking the pain crisis for attention. But unfortunately, that was my life and that was my reality. I knew most of the doctors and nurses at the various hospitals and clinics I visited by name. I became a surrogate daughter to them. They had consistently watched me struggle through my young life.

    I was elated when I began to mature as a young woman and started developing breasts. I was excited because I knew it was a matter of time before I became a young woman. Yes, I was looking forward to this period of my life because somewhere along the journey in growing up, I had heard a few people talk about the possibility of the frequency of pain crisis decreasing as I matured into young womanhood. I was looking forward to a time in my life when, I would not have as many pain crises as I was currently experiencing. Another reason I was excited about my development into a young woman was experiencing a menstrual cycle. This sounds silly, right? Well, at this point in life, most of my friends had been through it and it had become a topic of discussion on many occasions both at home and at school. My desire was to be able to share in that experience with my friends and be as normal as I possibly could. I felt the need to be a part of the experience and to feel like a young woman too. I wanted my hips to look curvy and my breasts bigger so that certain clothes would fit and look better on me. Little did I know these monthly menstrual cycles would turn out to be one of the major dreads in my life. An experience though exciting and a sign of maturity for most teenage girls, would turn out to be my most challenging and most dreadful time of the month. I would live to despise this part of my life for a very long time.

Finally, at sixteen years of age I experienced my first menstrual cycle. As expected, the first cycle was painful. Under the impression that subsequent cycles would be less painful; I was in for a rude awakening. Less painful cycle was certainly not the case for me. My cycle was never consistent; it was painful each and every month; and caused a great deal of discomfort. Every cycle was bound to put me into a pain crisis of some sort. Every single menstrual cycle! Of course some of the crisis was less painful than others and hence manageable at home. However, most of the time, my cycle would bring on painful crisis sending me into the hospital on many occasions. When on admission, the doctors would provide treatment to help ease the pain for a number of days. The pain would usually register in my lower back and legs and sometimes my chest area. This whole menstrual cycle experience was not exciting anymore. This womanhood experience was quickly turning into a dreadful one, month after month. I no longer looked forward to my cycles and often wished it would seize. Yet I also knew if I ever wanted to bear children of my own in the future, this process was a necessity in life to afford me that opportunity. When friends of mine had little or no issues during their cycles and talked about them so casually and nonchalantly, I was jealous and wished things were different for me.

    Through all this I managed to enjoy life as best as I could. I had a boyfriend or should I say boyfriends at various stages of my teenage life. I went to parties when my parents permitted and I had friends come hang out at home after school. I had lots of friends and had a great deal of fun and lots of great memories I will forever hold dear. At some point I begun to prepare to take the Standard Aptitude Test (SAT) and Test of English as a Foreign Language (TOEFL) in preparation to attend college in the United States of America (U.S.A). My scores for both the SAT and TOEFL were good and I was able to gain admission into several colleges in the U.S.A. I opted to attend George Mason University, Fairfax, Virginia, where I would be close to my older sister Pamela. The time to leave for college quickly came and even though the future was uncertain when it came to dealing with SCD, I hoped coming to the U.S.A. would be the best. I hoped this would be the best in terms of the availability of options in treatment for this disease and my parent's agreed with me.

Chapter 12

In August of 1995 I arrived in the U.S.A to join Pamela and Dennis, my older siblings. The plan was for me to return home to assist with the family business, after obtaining my bachelors degree. It was an opportunity provided to me by my parents to further my education outside of Ghana, experience another country and culture while exposing myself to things that will enhance my growth and maturity into adulthood. Coming to the U.S.A. was one of the best decisions my parents made for me especially when it comes to medical care. With my condition I needed the best medical resources available and they could not have picked a better place for me. I also needed to be close to family to have the support of people who knew me and knew of my struggle with SCD.

My decision to attend college in the U.S.A. was easy and by default since this was where my older siblings were. My older sister Pam had been the first to leave home to attend the Bradford School of Business in Pittsburg later transferring to George Mason University in Virginia. My brother Dennis followed 2 years later to Philadelphia attending the Temple University. Two years after Dennis left Ghana, it was my turn to embark on this journey too. By then, Pam had transferred from Pittsburg to Virginia. It was therefore the ideal situation for me. Pam was a great source of knowledge and support especially during this period of my transition. Both she and Dennis were of tremendous help, although Pam was my constant and unshakeable support system. She helped with the transition and exposure to college life. She was there when I was having difficulty adjusting to the new country, culture and its changing seasons. Pam was also there when I went into pain crisis for the first time here not knowing what to do without our parents. She stepped in and made sure I was taken care of. She was my compass in navigating this world that was so foreign to me at the time.

Clara joined us a year later. Like Pam and Dennis, she joined in providing the love and support I need. My parents and grandmother though thousands of miles away visited as often as they could. Even from afar, they also built a loving and supporting cocoon around me which helped me with facing the challenges that lay ahead. We had family and friends who also provided support in many different ways. Without them, I cannot imagine how my siblings and I would have made it. Whenever I was severely ill, Mom would drop everything she was dealing with back home to help care for me. Dad was always so supportive and understanding and without a doubt, he would always come through by making travel arrangements for her to be here within days. My siblings, extended family and friends had other obligations like school, work and other life's demands and as such could only help so much. There were times when Mom would spend months, sometimes a year in the US caring for me. Edward had to work to provide for us and as a result, he was unable to visit as frequently as Mom did. Occasionally he would visit for short periods of time as his job would allow.

Although I was the one that carried the SCD, it affected my family as a whole. Because of the unpredictability and the severity of the pain crisis; the complications that came with the disease; the strong medications I had to be on; among other things, my family always thought it was best to be around my siblings. As a result, I always lived with either Pam or Clara until recently. I was resigned to the fact that this was going to be my life. I accepted that and tried to live as normal a life as possible. Little did I know that God had a different plan and that there was going to be a pivotal moment in my future that would completely change my life.

Chapter 13

During my freshman year at George Mason University, I was enrolled under a program which was designed for international students to be connected with American families to aid in their transition into the culture. Through this program, I was connected with Ms. Fran Boyle who became not only my host Mom, but my surrogate Mom. Fran not only stood in for my parents during the difficult periods I was faced with, but also stood in as a surrogate Mom for all my siblings. Fran was and has continued to be a major support system for us. With her strength, dedication, love and most importantly prayers, we overcame not only the complications from SCD and numerous hospitalizations, but other major challenges and struggles.

Though finding my way to the U.S.A seemed like a great idea initially, over time, it seemed as though the winter months was not conducive for me. I was getting attacks more frequently than usual all year round, but especially during the winter months. At this point, not only was I worried about monthly pain crisis from my menstrual cycle; I was also worried about the bouts of pain that I was dealt with during the unpredictable and frequent weather changes. I was on admission at various hospitals in the D.C., Maryland and Virginia area quite frequently. Facilities like the INOVA Fairfax, Fairoaks, and Alexandria hospitals, as well as, the Howard University hospital were my home away from home of sorts. I was in and out of these medical facilities so often that I knew what the admissions routines and processes were in each hospital. The unpredictability and frequency of the pain crisis attacks made it difficult to have a normal college life. Unlike most college students my age, I could not find the time or the energy to attend parties, go out drinking, or engage in the fun my colleagues and peers enjoyed. One sip of any alcoholic beverage would put me into a crisis anyway. So I could not participate in that lifestyle even if I wanted to.

Also, the frequency and unpredictability disease made it challenging many times to keep up with course work. Thankfully I had professors who not only understood my situation, but were also very accommodating. They adjusted deadlines for me and schedules so I could catch up on my course work. During the spring semester of my sophomore year, I was so gravely ill that I had to withdraw from school. I returned the following semester. I was blessed with an internship with Harvey E. Johnson, CPA in Arlington, VA during my junior year in college. This internship overtime became a full-time job for me when I graduated from college. The owner of the firm and my former boss who is now deceased also became a father figure to me. Harvey was very understanding of my condition; very accommodating; and I never had to worry about having a job for as long as he lived. God placed such wonderful people in my life to make life a little easy on me and on my family.

In spite of all the hurdles I faced, I was able to graduate with a bachelor's degree in May of 2000. Considering everything I had gone through, it was a great accomplishment for me to be able to graduate college. As I walked up to receive my diploma, I became overwhelmed with a feeling of accomplishment that filled my heart with joy and my eyes with tears from the fulfillment I was feeling. Most of all, I also had a job lined up. What more could I ask for, I thought to myself. I had grown to accept the fact that I had been dealt this hand and was forging my way through life by figuring out a way to juggle, life, work and living with SCD. At the time I thought SCD was the only medical condition I had to face. I was willing to figure out a way to live life with this disease.

Chapter 14

One beautiful morning in the spring of 2003, my younger sister Clara asked me to accompany her to Washington D.C. District court to follow up on a case she was researching on. I dressed up that morning in a lovely print skirt and a white crisp blouse and downed on a pair of heels. The court visit was a success and on our way back, as I crossed a street in D.C. I twisted my left ankle and almost fell. I did not think anything of it and assumed it was the two-inch heel that had gotten in the way somehow. Later on that day while I was taking a shower, my left leg felt weakened and I almost fell in the shower. I realized although I could bear weight on that particular leg, it felt weak and funny. That got me thinking about the day's events and I began to worry. By night time I was experiencing a weakness in the whole of my left leg. I was worried and decided to get it checked out. My sisters Pam and Clara accompanied me to the Alexandria Hospital Emergency Room that evening.

Upon probing and testing and answering many questions, with my history of Sickle Cell Anemia, the initial thought that it was the occurrence of a Stroke. At some point the idea of my symptoms being those of Bell's palsy came up. These different diagnoses being thrown out there were not only confusing, but frightening. How and why could this be happening to me? Finally after further extensive tests which consisted of a spinal tap and blood work among others, I was diagnosed with Multiple Sclerosis

(MS). I was dealt the devastating blow of having Multiple Sclerosis. What the HECK? My sisters and I thought? That was the first time we had all heard of this disease. What did those words mean and how was that going to impact my life? How could I have Multiple Sclerosis on top of Sickle Cell Disease? This was mind-blowing, to say the least. This was one of the most difficult and wearisome times of my life. It was a difficult time for me and for my family. I was angry. Yes, I was angry at the world and I was angry at God. How could He allow this to happen to me? What had I ever done wrong in life to be handed such a blow?

After learning about the MS diagnosis and what I was faced with in addition to what I was dealing with already, I did and could not fathom how I was going to live through life like this. I could not imagine life like this. I was upset, frustrated and became depressed. I was sad. How could this happen to me? Was my suffering with SCD not enough? What had I done to deserve this? Why me? My questions were endless. I had been asking God to heal me for years and He had not. And I was at a point in life where I had accepted living with SCD. But for MS to be added onto that was indeed a situation that put me into a tailspin and into depression. I can honestly say the first year after diagnosis was the most difficult. I eventually embraced it and resigned myself to the fact that this was the hand I had been dealt and was unwillingly going to live with it the best way I could with the support of my family, friends and medication. For years I was on Copaxone and was self administering my daily shots of the medication. Through all these difficult times, God gave me strength.

Chapter 15

Shortly after my diagnosis with MS, we learned about the National Institutes of Health (NIH). We read about some of the research studies and protocols the NIH offered for various conditions including Sickle Cell Disease. The main purpose of these research studies is to provide knowledge and insights into different conditions which in turn allow the medical team to formulate and implement processes and procedures to help care for patients. These research studies and protocols are available to help both patients and researchers develop strategies beneficial to all. Prior to educating ourselves on what these studies involves and making an informed decision to be part of a research study, the thought of being part of a research study/protocol sounded frightening. It was frightening because we were imagining the worst. Our thought process was that we would be used as "lab rats". We did not view being part of a study as being beneficial to the participant, the NIH, as well as other patients. We had tunnel vision at the time.

We pondered over this for a period of time and eventually made the decision to visit NIH to learn more about their research studies and protocols. The visit was enlightening and helped abate the fears and concerns we had. A few months after our initial visit to NIH, Clara and I enrolled in one of their protocols for SCD. We were introduced at the time to the new drug for SCD disease which was Hydroxy Urea. The team at NIH closely monitored us while on this medication. Over time, the frequency of the pain crisis decreased. While this was good news, I was still dealing with the occasional MS flare ups. But overall, things seemed to have calmed down somewhat for me. I thought I was home free and was accepting to live my life this way. In my mind, the few pain crises were something I could accept and embrace for the rest of my life.

After a few years of being on Hydorxy Urea, things changed. The medication was not being as effective as it had been in the past. My body was not responding to this treatment anymore. Thus the medical team took me off the medication although I still remained under their care on another protocol. The pain crises became so frequent again. Each pain crisis that led to an emergency room visit or hospitalization meant that I would need intravenous fluids, both oral and intravenous medications and a possible blood transfusion(s). Overtime my veins got tired and were not cooperating effectively in the administering of IV care anymore. It became difficult for my veins to be accessed when in crisis and needed a quick administering of IV care. A medi-port had to be inserted in my chest to aid this process. The purpose of this medi-port was to aid in the quick, reliable and consistent administration of medication and IV fluids during pain crises. With this medi-port I was assured of getting the treatment I needed for faster pain relief. Even though its purpose was to help me, I despised having this port sitting on my chest. It was another reminder to myself and to others of how sick I was. There was no way I could hide being sick from people. With this port being so obvious, there was no way I could pretend I was a "normal" person. Those that were not familiar with it would ask questions, which in turn made me more and more self conscious.

As most Sickle Cell patients can attest, the pain crisis can be excruciating and intense. The pain attacks could manifest at any given day, place or time. However, overtime, there were certain activities that I knew would put me into crisis. Some of these activities included swimming or walking briskly for a long period of time and not keeping myself hydrated. Therefore I stayed away from them. The intensity of the pain varied and that determined the pain management regimen I used. With the less intense pain I was able to manage the pain at home with medications like prescription strength Ibuprofen and fluids. On the other hand, I treated the more severe pain with controlled substances such as Dilaudid, Percocet or Oxycontin. For extremely severe pain, I would go into the hospital where doctors would administer IV pain medication such as morphine, IV Antibiotics (if necessary) with IV fluids. Dealing with this disease for so many years allowed me to know my body and know when to make the decision of either going into the hospital or managing the pain at home.

The interference and disruption of living my life from SCD was starting to take a major toll on me. I could no longer find strength in my faith. Getting into crises almost every month with my menstrual cycles, missing work, missing activities, and missing life in general put me into depression. Although I did not acknowledge I was in a depressed state at the time, my family and doctors saw the depression and knew I needed help. I did not see the downward spiral I was in. On many occasions, I felt as though life was not worth living anymore. I watched my friends and my siblings live their lives. Unlike them, my life was always being interrupted by these two diseases and I did not and could see a way out. How could I see a way out when my days were clouded with pain and numbness. Ingesting countless medications to treat the pain and giving myself shots to treat my MS became my routine. How could I see a way out when holding a full time job was a struggle? How could I see a way out and live a productive life with all these challenges coming at me?

Chapter 16

Due to the numerous pain crises over the years, I developed Avascular Necrosis (AVN) in both shoulders and hips. This diagnosis came about after I begun to experience pain in my shoulders which also subsequently made it difficult to use my arms. Many individuals with SCD also suffer from the long-term consequences of vaso-occlusive pain episodes in the musculoskeletal system, such as AVN. This often leads to a chronic state of pain in addition to the more acute painful episodes. Although the pain was severe mainly in the right shoulder, mobility in both shoulders was limited. It was painful reaching out to grab something or whenever attempted to put on my clothes. Initially, the pain I experienced was not intense; however, it worsened over time, becoming so severe that no amount of pain medication would ease the pain. And that was when I was diagnosed with AVN as the x-rays revealed the extent of the damage. It was difficult doing simple things like opening the door of a vehicle to get out some days. How can I live like this I thought many nights? I wanted to end it all many days.

I was placed on medications like Oxycontin, and Neurontin among others to help alleviate some of the pain. Yet I could not find relief. Initially I was using Oxycontin to help ease the pain. But there came point when Oxycontin helped provide a relief and also an escape from the pain I was living in. That was, the dark cloud of pain and frustration of my life. Soon I was taking narcotic pain medicine not only to numb the crises and pain from AVN, but to also numb the emotional pain I was in. Yes, I was in an emotional pain that was not easily discernible to the naked eye. I was in an emotional pain that only I knew existed. I was depressed and soon my vision and thoughts became blurred. My vision, thoughts and reality were all the same. I was unable to distinguish between when I was taking narcotics for pain versus when I was taking it just to escape my reality. My reality was facing life constantly in pain. The excruciating pain from AVN, the pain from the Sickle Cell crisis; the numbness in parts of my body from MS, among other complications caused me to spiral into a dark hole. Though the MS flare up was not painful, it was still a reason to take narcotics to escape. The thought of not living a normal and productive life made me seek an avenue to escape my reality. The only avenue I knew at the time was to self medicate with narcotics. I could not see or think of anything positive in my life. Those big brown almond shaped eyes shed many tears of pain. These tears were from the frustration of living in constant pain. When will all it end? I often wondered. When will I be free? Will I ever get relief? Not short-term relief from pain medicine, but long-term relief which is what I hoped for. These were some of the questions that went through my mind.

My point of escape became narcotics even when I did not need them. Often times I would take extra doses of the pain medicine at night with the hopes of falling into a sound sleep and not waking up the next morning. I would take extra doses of various narcotics hoping and praying that I would not wake up to face another day like this. Yes, that is how low I felt. I wanted to escape this world on many nights. In my eyes, this life was not worth living. I wanted to escape and be free. Yes, free of the misery and the pain I was in. God being the God He is, never allowed any of my attempts at suicide to work. God knew what he was about to do and the plans He had for me. Somehow He stood in the way of my attempt to leave this world because He knew that was not a part of His plan for me. In hindsight I am so happy that none of those attempts worked. I am happy because I am now living my best life ever. I have not accomplished my purpose in this life. The work He has for me on this earth has not been completed yet.

    The need for narcotics turned me into a different person. The addiction to pain medicine turned me into a person I am not proud of. The addiction turned me into a liar and a thief. I would steal pain medicine from my sister Clara who also needed it for her pain management and even when caught I'd lie about it. It changed me to engage in behaviors, I now cannot fathom. I almost always found a reason to stay home when there was an event the whole family was expected to attend. I began lying to my family I was in pain just so I could stay home and wallow in the depression that was consuming me. I was not a pleasant person to be around. My self-esteem was as low as it could get. I forced myself daily to put a smile on my face and pretend I was happy just so my family and friends would think I was alright and get off my back. It was the only way I could hide the pain I was in. I tried my best to pretend I was happy to all the people around me.

Even though I pretended to have one, I had no confidence in myself. I always felt sorry for myself; I always felt like a victim; and took everything personal. I was unhappy and projected it unto others, especially those closest to me.. My family was bearing the brunt of my anger and frustration. Although they continued to love and support me I still felt so alone. I could be in the middle of a crowded room and still felt alone. Whenever I was approached by doctors, nurses and family about my addiction, I would deny it. Like any addict, I could never admit nor accept I was an addict although my gut feeling told me so. It was a catch twenty two for me. I needed the medication for pain and so it was difficult for my team of doctors to refuse to provide me with any. Yet, on the other hand, this same medication that was to relive my pain was serving my addiction. Thankfully the medical team implemented various systems to help with the addiction.

The team developed a plan to help me deal with this problem by implementing a system of accountability. The initial plan was to allow me to have a specific number of pills for a period of time. If the pills run out before they were scheduled to be refilled, I would have to explain why. Another plan put in place was for my mother or one of my sisters to be in charge of dispensing the pain medication. I was not allowed to keep them as I did previously. It was entrusted to my sisters the goal of which was to ensure accountability and curtail my addiction. While this plan was for my good, I did not see it that way. Knowing their habits and tendencies, I would figure out where they hid the medication and would occasionally steal some. I tried to fight the plan and came up with so many excuses and reasons why I needed the medication so frequently or needed to be in control of it. Thankfully the team would not budge. The team did everything they could to help me through this.

Chapter 17

In the spring of 2004, due to complications from a blood transfusion as a result of the development of antibodies in my body, I went into a Coma. At the time, I went into the coma, I was not only having a pain crisis, but I was also experiencing an MS flare up. I fell into the Coma and was in it for six days. It was a petrifying time for my family. It was a difficult time because no one could tell how this would play out. No one could tell what the outcome would be. Would I ever recover? And if so when? Would I be a different person? What would the prognosis be? The questions were endless. While in the ICU, my family never left my side. They made sure there was always someone with me, not because they did not trust the team, but because they wanted me to see a familiar face whenever I came to. My mother especially kept a vigil by my bed side. She looked on daily as doctors and nurses came to my bed side changing tubes, administering medications of various kinds. She looked on as the doctors discussed my condition and relay the information to her. She was gravely concerned.

My Mom asked questions and sought answers from them for her sanity and peace of mind. The medical team encouraged my family to talk to me even during this time. They encouraged this because they believed even in Coma; a patient could still hear the voice of their loved ones. My mother who is one of the strongest women I know would talk to me on a daily basis. Even in my

Comatose state, she would tell me what was going on with my siblings, she would tell me to keep fighting and come back to the love that was waiting for me. My mother says she and my siblings continued to encourage me to keep fighting daily and prayed God would work His continued miracle. Through all my health struggles, I never once saw my mother shed a tear. Her tears were shed in the presence of God, in prayer and supplication to God for healing. Never in my presence did I see her or my Dad cry in frustration or sadness. All they wanted was for me to fight.

    On the sixth day of being in the Coma, I woke up like I had just been in a deep sleep. I woke up to the sound of my mother's voice that day. She had been in the middle of sharing with me stories about one of my siblings when she noticed movement. She paused and asked if I wanted a drink of water. I reacted and said yes. She offered me a sip of water and I opened my eyes after that. She was so happy and excited and yet unsure of what to think or do. She pressed the call bell and alerted my nurse I had opened my eyes. My nurse came rushing to the room as she called the doctor on call to inform them of the news. As my eyes assessed and focused on my surroundings, I saw the joy and relief on not only my Mom face, but that of the medical team in whose care I was. This day was yet another day of one of the miracles God worked in my life.

Coming out of this Coma was not the end of this hurdle. I spent a few more weeks in this facility and finally made it home. I spent a few weeks at home to fully recover and eventually returned to my daily routine. The thought of having gone through this experience impacted me in the sense that I felt God's strength more than ever. I felt He was with me no matter what. Although it was very traumatic experience, it also taught me that life is indeed too short and that tomorrow is not promised to anyone.

I lived my life as normal as I possibly could. I lived by engaging in things young adults engage in. That is work, friends, parties, boyfriends and different responsibilities presented in life. I dealt with them in the best way I could and in the best way my health would allow me to.

Chapter 18

Though I am unsure where or how to begin on the topic of relationships, I will start off by sharing how I often dealt with my relationships. I was generally open in all my relationships about my medical status especially the SCD. I always shared this information with whomever I dated that I had Sickle Cell Disease and Multiple Sclerosis. It was never a secret. I was open and honest about it. I believed and still believe honesty is a great foundation for a successful relationship. The revelation that I had SCD, more often than not, turned the gentlemen away instead. My approach was to be transparent, but it almost always backfired on me. I do not hold any anger, resentment, or regret against any of the gentlemen I dated as I would probably have reacted in the same manner had the tables been turned.

Even though people know of Sickle Cell Disease, most think it is a death sentence and in ignorance assume people with this disease have a short span of life; are unable to hold jobs; are drug addicts; unable to have kids; unable to live productive lives; and the list goes on. Society carries a stigma about individuals with SCD. Granted, it is a challenging disease, yet, there are many sickle cell patients who have lived and continue to live productive lives. I know of sickle cell patients who have managed to navigate through life successfully although not without difficulty. I believe the negative reactions are a result of hearsay and from the fear of the unknown. Instead of understanding that each patient is different and hence each outcome is also different, people form assumptions rather than making judgments on an individual basis.

At one point, I was to get engaged to a great guy I had met through a mutual friend. At the beginning I could sense his mother's anxiety and hesitation with the fact that I had SCD. Yet when I had asked him about it, he assured me that his mind was made up about moving forward with the engagement. That was what he led me to believe. I had been an open book from the beginning sharing with him the challenges I've had and continue to face. About a month before the traditional engagement was to take place, I checked in with him on the status of the dowry, a customary rite practiced in the Ghanaian culture. Generally, the bride-to-be's family provides the groom with a list of items to provide as part of the dowry. The presentation of these items and a ring at the ceremony and in the presence of family and friends is part of the engagement ceremony. It was then that he revealed to me that he had a change of mind about moving forward with the ceremony. He did not want to proceed with the engagement after all. The reason for this decision was because his Mother was not comfortable with his decision to marry me. His mother was concerned with me becoming a burden to her son. What a shock that was. The shock was not about how his mother felt about my condition, as I already knew how she felt, rather the shock was from him agreeing to listen to the negative things his mother believed about me and the fact that he had the nerve to convey that to me. But I guess as an obedient and respectful son, he had to do as his mother requested.

His mother strongly felt I would live a short life due to SCD and or become a burden to her son. She also felt; I would not be able to bear children for her son; I would always be sick and become a burden to him. His mother felt her son could do better and should not proceed with the engagement. He agreed with his mother and therefore broke off the engagement. So we went our separate ways and life went on. You can only imagine how those words made me feel. I was depressed, angry, and hurt to the core. Not only did I not see this coming, but for this guy and his mother to think this of me, hurt me to the core resulting in depression and hate. Not only did I hate my life at this point, but I also hated them until I learned to forgive them. I had to forgive them to do away with the hatred I harbored towards them.

By the time I was diagnosed with MS, I did not even want a boyfriend. I was so angry and depressed that sharing my life with a partner was the last thing I could think off. It was difficult enough finding a partner with having SCD. Imagine how difficult it would be announcing to a potential partner I was dealing with SCD and MS. I am sure my family will tell you I was neither the nicest nor the happiest person to be around for most of the time during the period after my MS diagnosis. After the cancellation of my engagement, I took on life one day at a time and often prayed to God to allow me to find a mate who would embrace me with all my challenges.

Chapter 19

In 2009, I was approached by my doctors at NIH with the idea of bone marrow transplantation. This idea sounded so good to me that with faith and the expertise of some great doctors, it changed my life. Out of concern by the doctors and with the hope of improving my quality of life, they felt this would be an impactful option to consider. Being one of their sickest patients over the last few years, observing me on admission multiple times a month with severe sickle cell crises or an MS flared up, the medical team was concerned and wanted to take this opportunity to help me obtain a better quality of life. I was approached with the idea of Stem Cell Transplant being a possible cure for Sickle Cell Anemia. The team informed me this procedure was still in its experimental stages and there was no guarantee it would be a success. This was exciting news and I agreed almost immediately having not heard the details involved.

Although I had heard of Stem Cell transplant being a potential cure for SCD, I never thought I would see the day where such an opportunity would be made available to me. I never imagined I would even be considered a viable candidate for a procedure like this. My mindset was that there was nothing medically that could be done to improve my life. Nothing could possibly turn things around for me. Mentally I had placed a lid on what God could do as far as my health was concerned. Intellectually I had placed a limitation on God and assumed God was no longer performing the miracles He used to perform. I was of the mindset that God had completed his task of working miracles due to our sinful nature in this age and time. Yes, this was my mind set. After all, I had been praying for years for healing and healing had never come. I had shed many tears day and night requesting God to relieve me of this burden and nothing had changed. Therefore decidedly I had placed a limit on what He could do at this point in my life. I never looked at my request as one that could be answered in God's time. I wanted my prayers answered immediately at the time. And when God had not answered them as I had hoped, I begun to settle and place limitations on my healing. It had been almost thirty-six years after all and there was no way I would ever be cured. It was not possible at all I thought

    Here I was being presented with an opportunity that could possibly change things for the better. Little did I know that God was going to be using science and a great medical team to provide the answer to my petition. He was ready to move after thirty-six years of prayer and supplication. God had heard my cries after all. He had heard them all and was ready in His timing to change my situation. He needed me to surrender and put my complete trust in Him. He needed me to be in a place where my faith in Him was stronger than ever. He wanted me to mature in faith and give Him control by surrendering. After the initial conversation regarding the transplant and agreeing to do it, it took several months to prepare not only my body, but my mind and also to strengthen my faith for this procedure. Even though I was advised about the major potential risks involved in this process, God gave me a faith I had never had before. I believed from the beginning that Stem Cell Transplant was my door to walk out of the "tunnel" I was in. I believed it would work for me even when others thought otherwise. And I thank God for giving me such strong conviction and faith about this.

I discussed this opportunity with very close family members. Though worried about the possible complications that could develop from the procedure, they were equally excited about the opportunity and immediately backed me up in faith and through their actions. We all had questions and some concerns. At the same time they were excited about what that possibility could bring. We consulted with the team of doctors when we needed to and they did their best to address our concerns. My parents and siblings supported me in my decision to undergo the procedure. The next step after making my decision was to find a match/donor. We set out to find a match and undergo preparation for the transplant and this process was called the HLA typing screening which took several months. The process included the HLA typing screens which was required of my parents; as well as, Pam, Dennis and Clara. It took about a year to complete the testing for a match and ensuring I was in a good place mentally and physically. The team decided my mother was a safe and perfect match.

During this preparation period, I never wavered in faith nor doubted this procedure would work. My mother was over the moon when testing had revealed she was a better match for me. Being a match and a donor for me was an opportunity Mom would not pass even if she could. This was the opportunity to help relieve me off some of the pain as she had always wished. It was a moment she had been waiting for. She was advised on how painful the process of preparing her body to generate excess bone marrow for harvest would be. Yet she was determined and willing to do anything she could. My mother would not have it any other way. This confirmed her love for me.

The cells were harvested from my mom about two weeks before the Haplotransplant actually took place. It was an exciting time. I was ready and anxious to undergo this process that had the potential to change my life. I was yearning to undertake this transformative process. My family and I prepared for the procedure by immersing ourselves in prayer and with the support of our church family and friends. We made the decision not to share the details of this upcoming procedure with many of people until it was completely over. The uncertainty of this daunting undertaking was petrifying enough that we needed to stay prayed up and positive. Although we had faith and trust in God, we did not know what to expect during the process and what the outcome would be. There were many uncertainties ahead and keeping it intimate and rather immersing ourselves in prayer and in God's guidance and direction was what we thought was best.

Chapter 20

On November 8th of 2010, I went on admission at the National Institute of Health in Bethesda, Maryland. I checked in fully aware of what was to come. I was anxious yet excited! I was very excited about the possibilities to come. God had given me a strong resolve I had never had before. Although I was aware of the chances of this transplant not being a success, I had a strong conviction it would all work out for His sake. I had been informed this journey would not be an easy one. In fact, I had been informed there was a possibility I could encounter complications which could potentially put me in a worse medical condition than I already was in. Yet, that did not faze me. I had faith this transplant would work and I never focused on any of the other possible outcomes; and I thank God for giving me such faith. Nothing was going to cause me to fear or even allow me to think the possibility of this procedure not working. As I told my family, even if this meant experiencing a pain free life for just a day it would be worth it.

When I checked in on November 8th, I was expected to spend approximately three months there as I had been previously advised. The next few days after check in were focused on preparing me to receive the cells harvested a few weeks earlier. I received a low dose of chemo and a low dose of total body radiation during this initial period. The purpose of this part of the transplant process was to suppress my immune system and allow my body to be receptive when the "foreign" cells were administered.

This would reduce the chance of rejection. Days after chemo and radiation my hair began to fall out as expected. Although I was aware the hair loss was an imminent part of the procedure, I just was not prepared for it. One morning, I was taken by shock when I felt chunks of my hair in the palm of my hand as I run my hands through my hair. I began to cry. Yes, I cried, it was so real I did not know what to think of it. My medical team helped me deal with it by offering the services of a barber. I agreed to it immediately as this felt like taking control by having it cut instead of watch the remaining hair slowly fall out. In fact, it helped me handle the hair loss better.

During this time, the staff, doctors and nurses treated my family and I with dignity and respect. They all made us especially me very comfortable during my stay. I was provided with a variety of resources to while away the time. I had access to priests, a library, a gym and a host of other amenities that helped make my stay there a little easy and feel as normal as possible. The team of doctors and nurses kept me and my family informed every step of the way. They kept us up to date on all test results, procedures and/or medication administered. They always set expectations. Over time, I began to feel and see changes in my body. I lost my appetite for food and lost weight as time progressed. But this was just the beginning. Knowing what a long road was ahead for me, I braced myself and surrounded myself with music, prayers, love and support of hospital staff and most importantly my family. I kept in touch via phone with those who could not be physically present with me. I took it one day at a time.

Chapter 21

For a long period of time I had longed for my healing. In fact I had been at the Pool of Bethesda for over thirty-seven years and watched others get their healing. I had seen others receive their breakthrough and often wondered when mine would occur. The edge of the pool had been my seat for an extensive period of time. I was just unable to push myself into it when it was stirred. My relief and my healing had been elusive. No matter how hard I prayed, how well I ate, how well hydrated myself, how willing and open I was to trying new medications, etc.; my healing never came. When the pool was stirred, others jumped in before I could gather myself to jump in. Others moved faster by responding well to various treatments. They jumped in faster than I could.

There were multiple breakthrough attempts at the pool but somehow, none of them seemed to work for me. In an effort to help me manage Sickle Cell Disease (SCD), Multiple Sclerosis (MS), and the other health conditions I faced, my doctors had tried various treatments in terms of medications, but none of which had been effective in the long-term. I also tried non-conventional approaches like acupuncture and reike to manage my pain. I tried them all and at my pool of Bethesda, my attempts were fruitless. As much as I tried, I could not jump in the pool to cleanse myself of my illnesses. I did not have the energy to push myself to look beyond my circumstances. I did not have the faith I needed to help give me a lift to jump in. I was focused on the wrong things. I did not look at my circumstance from a place of victory. I did not see my healing as ever being possible. I was crippled by the "woe is me" mentality. In the end when I could see, feel and taste my healing; and when God's time was right, I finally received what I had been praying for. God's timing is and was the best for me. When I had hope, and exercised faith, God stepped in and I was about to undergo a procedure which I believed would bring me the long-term relief I had always longed for.

According to one of the doctors, the impetus to inform me of this experimental procedure was due to the fact that she saw an extremely difficult life ahead of me. With time, complications from Sickle Cell Disease and Multiple Sclerosis had the potential to make my life complicated, challenging and possibly a short one. It was difficult for the team to watch me come to their facility so frequently. They were concerned not only at the frequency, but at the level of pain I was dealing with. The quantities and dosage of pain medications I needed to alleviate the pain, and the number of blood transfusions, were also of great concern. The future looked grim for me from their point of view if my life continued in this direction.

November 18th, 2010 was the day of my rebirth. This was the day my life would change forever. I had been told the cells would be administered on this day and my family and I had continued to engage in immense prayer asking God to facilitate this process and show His mighty hand. My host Mom Fran Boyle who had been by my side every step of the way since I arrived in the US was in serious prayer with her prayer warriors. I could see the joy in Fran's eyes as this day approached. At approximately 8 am on this day, the cells harvested from my Mom, were administered. These cells were the cells that would turn my life upside down in a positive way. The cells were administered very slowly intravenously. The cells were administered over several hours. I lay in my hospital bed and watched the cells slowly make their way into my veins. I watched the IV tube slowly fill up with the stem cells. I could feel the excitement and fear in me grow at the same time. I was monitored very closely as the cells were administered. They ran a series of tests and procedures that revealed how my body was responding to the new cells. This process was very tough. I had a long road ahead of me.

The excitement was from the desire to be rid of the SCD and to live a "normal" productive life. The hint of fear was from the uncertainty that came with embarking on this life changing journey. I had watched not only my siblings but my friends and colleagues live life to the fullest. They did things I had wished for so long I could do. In my eyes they could engage in any activity they wanted and not have to worry about that activity causing them to go into painful crises. They could pick up and go out of town and not worry about having adequate and sufficient pain medication with them.

They never had to take time off work due to frequent hospital stay. They never had to play catch up in any area of their lives. This is what I had experienced for so long. This is how I had lived for so long and I was tired of it.

The doctors and nurses had a major endeavor on their hands yet they were all up for the challenge. They had carefully analyzed and considered previous research data; and made changes and adjustments where necessary in terms of their approach with the procedure. They had strategized for months and considered different scenarios and what their approach would be. This was a daunting undertaking. After all I was their fourth Haplo-identical transplant case and this particular transplant approach was quite new at the time. The team had not experienced any success in the three cases they had worked on previously. This procedure was not new to them; however, it was still daunting and filled with many uncertainties. While it was the desire of the team to rid me off this debilitating disease, the possibility of the procedure resulting in complications and potentially put my health and life in a more complicated situation was of great concern to them. This caused many on the team some sleepless nights. The last thing they wanted was to further decrease my quality of life. They hoped my case would be a success and give me a chance to live a better quality of life. This would also be a sign of encouragement to the world that progress was being made towards finding a cure for Sickle Cell Disease. The team hoped my case would be a success that would bring hope to patients.

Chapter 22

On December 7th 2010, after being in the hospital for almost a month, my test results confirmed I had 99% of the donor cells. This basically meant that I had engrafted. The medical team felt very confident at that point this transplant was a success. They were extremely overjoyed at the positive outcome of this challenging task. Each and every reaction my body manifested after each drug or treatment was exactly what the team had expected and had hoped for. The weight loss, loss of appetite, mucositis, hair loss, etc., were exactly what was expected to occur. No experience had deviated from the script, and this was very exciting and reassuring. In fact this was awesome!!! After keeping a close eye on me for a few more weeks, I was released to go home. After being in the hospital for approximately six weeks, I was finally discharged under very strict guidelines.

I felt weak and tired, yet optimistic about the weeks ahead. Although I was feeling great about SCD being cured, I still had a long road ahead of me. The fight was not over for me just yet. I was still under close observation and followed up with weekly appointments for months. The NHLBI department made provisions for me to get a couple of wigs to wear to help me get back to being my old self. I was required to wear a mask as a protection from infections. I was advised to wash my hands frequently and I was also to stay away from crowded places initially. Leaving the hospital with these instructions seemed as though they would be difficult to follow. However, knowing the fight for my life was not yet over, I had no choice but to follow the directions of my doctors to make this a success. My family and friends supported me through this process. Eventually the weekly appointments turned to monthly, and then to twice a year. I finally thought to myself, I am home, free of SCD and I thank God for bringing me this far. For about a year after the transplant, I had to make some adjustments in my life and I could not have done it without my support system - family and friends. They were my rock.

Chapter 23

My neurologist also confirmed I had been cured of Multiple Sclerosis after about year post transplant. I was overwhelmed with joy. I had received my healing, I thought to myself. I have been cured of two diseases considered to be incurable, SCD and MS. I consider myself as blessed to have been given a new lease on life. Not very many people get such an opportunity. And that is how God works, I thought to myself. He works when you least expect Him to. He has revealed His glory again.

In fact, since the transplant, life had been amazingly good. I was experiencing my BEST life ever. For once in my life, I felt normal. I felt normal in the sense that, I was living my life to the fullest without having to worry about pain crises or an MS attack. I was able to go to work every day and if I missed work it was because I was on vacation and not because I was sick or on admission in the hospital. I was finally driving and own my own car. I was also living on my own and not physically or financially dependent on anyone as I had been in the past. I was finally able to engage in the regular activities of life without having to worry about going into pain crisis or having an MS flare-up. By this time, I had become a speaker and an inspiration to many who heard my story. I shared the story of my healing through speaking engagements at the NIH and through my local chapter of the Sickle Cell Association. I was called on by many to share and encourage others with my story. I felt liberated and free. Little did I know life would throw another challenge at me.

In November of 2015, I underwent my routine annual check-up at the NIH, after which I went home thinking everything was fine. My annual check-up usually consists of a brain scan, bone scan, and extensive blood work among others. Everything went smoothly during the testing, and I recall feeling pretty confident and thinking nothing was out of the ordinary. In my mind, I thought everything had gone wonderfully well. After all I looked good and most importantly I felt great. In fact, I was feeling better than I had felt in years and was in the best shape I had ever been. I was exercising regularly by walking a couple of miles a day, eating healthy meals, and had even managed to get to an ideal weight at that particular point of my life. My list of medications had reduced drastically, and life could not have been better. I was on cloud nine and was not expecting this visit to reveal anything different from the last. I was upbeat and excited about life and the new possibilities that lay ahead. Work was going great. At this point in time, I had managed to maintain a full time job that carried with it some long hours and stressful days. My relationship with God was even stronger than it was before. I had even rededicated my life to God earlier that month in a public ceremony at the Strong Tower Church here in Fredericksburg, Virginia. I had great friends and a current member of the church serving as s part of the hospitality team. I was thriving in life.

A few days after this appointment, I received a call from my doctor at NIH one morning that got me baffled. During the phone conversation, she advised me she had seen what she believed to be blood clots in my brain. She believed there were three brain aneurysms and that was of great concern to her and the medical team. Her suggestion was for me to see a Neurosurgeon as soon as possible. I was in shock during this phone conversation, that frankly I could not recall a lot of the details she had provided after I hung up. Instead what I do remember from the conversation were blood clots and seeing a neurosurgeon. After getting off the phone, I sat quietly, and took a few moments to process this information. A lot of questions went through my mind. "What does this mean?" and "How big were the clots?" and "What if they rupture?" and "Will I die?" and "How was this going to impact my life?" and "Did I come this far to die?" and "How did these clots develop?"

It was beginning to seem as though I could not catch a break! The old thoughts and anxiety I used to have before the transplant resurfaced. Once again, fear and worry wanted to take over my life. Why is there always something medically wrong with me, I thought to myself. Why did I come this far to face another challenge? Was this "stumbling block" going to prevent me from living the normal and productive life I was just getting used to?

Yes, there were unending questions that run through my mind. I had to remind myself of my moments of hope. I reminded myself of my blessings and the fact that my wish of living a day without pain had come true. In fact, I had been pain free for several years. I then made a decision to leave it all in God's hands. Although I was worried and scared, I decided to trust God wherever this would lead. It was God who had brought me this far. He had seen me through many trials therefore I knew He would see me through this one too. I immediately reminded myself of God's greatness, as I had experienced it firsthand. I had seen it manifest in so many ways and in varying areas of my life. I was not going down without a fight. I was not going through this cowardly. No, I had a God to whom nothing is impossible. I resolved to fight this with a stronger faith and a greater reliance on God. And I did.

My sisters were equally shocked when I came home and shared the news with them. I called my parents and brother to break the news to them as well. They all felt blindsided by this news and had a ton of questions just like I did. My family was supportive and encouraging as they have always been. We agreed not to rush to any conclusions, but rather focus on scheduling an appointment with the neurosurgeon as soon as possible to obtain more detailed information. While I waited to get an appointment, we agreed to engage in continued prayers and trust God through this. I do not know what I would have done through all of this without the love and support of my family and friends.

My team at NIH provided me with the name of a neurosurgeon at John Hopkins Hospital, who happened to be one of the best in the country. He was also one of the world's leaders in the endovascular treatment of cerebral aneurysms. This reminded me of how blessed I was to even have the opportunity to be under his care. The neurosurgeon ordered additional tests, one of them being an angiogram which revealed the clots were bigger and also that there were actually five of them and not three as originally thought. Yes, five of them!!! There were two aneurysms at the back of each eye and one aneurysm at the base of my brain. The aneurysms varied from 4.2 mm to 5.8 mm in size. The most interesting thing is, I was not experiencing any symptoms whatsoever. I was advised these needed to be taken care off right away to avoid the possibility of the clots rupturing. There was the potential for major complications or even death if any of them should rapture.

Mostly known for his expertise in the use of innovative flow-diverting stents and endovascular flow disrupters for treatment of cerebral aneurysms, the neurosurgeon was amazed by the fact that I was walking around with five aneurysms in my brain with no symptoms. He informed me of how serious and potentially life threatening these could be should they rupture. It was then, that I realized God's greatness and why He still had me breathing. That confirmed for me my purpose on this earth. I was blessed to have been directed into the hands of this doctor who would take care of these monsters in my brain. Yes I felt like the aneurysms were monsters that did not belong there. These aneurysms could have been developed as a result of my history with Sickle Cell Disease or family history. In 2016, I underwent three different embolization procedures over a period of three months to take care of the clots. By the Grace of God all three procedures went well. Today I am still alive and I do not exhibit any signs of this event ever taking place. He redeemed Himself again. I have continued in the care of my medical team at the NIH and John Hopkins as recommended.

Chapter 24

It has been almost eight years since I underwent this groundbreaking procedure and since the success of the transplant, my life has changed. My life has changed in that I have not experienced a single pain crisis and/or MS flare-up since. Today, I am able to engage in activities I could not engage in before the transplant. I went back to work eventually and got in the everyday grind that comes with the territory.

It was not the end of my medical trials. I began experiencing pain post transplant from the AVN in both shoulders and hips. The damage resulting from AVN is one that could not be reversed or cured by the transplant. Living with Sickle Cell Disease for all those years did cause some damage to my joints which is the result of atrophy of the bones in my joints. Overtime, the pain in my right hip worsened; making it painful to move. I knew what this meant because I had been told years earlier that subsequently I would need to have a hip replacement to fix the problem. On April 19th, 2017, I had a total hip replacement surgery on my right hip. Leading up to the surgery, I was informed I would have to stop taking Sirolimus which is the immunosuppressant drug that was keeping my old cell, that is, sickle cell disease at bay. I was advised to stop taking this medication five days before surgery and stay off it after surgery until I was cleared before I could go back on it. The reason for this plan of action was due to the fact that when one gets a wound while on the immunosuppressant drug, the wound takes a longer to heal. Therefore to ensure the wound would heal quickly, I had to come off the drug. This also meant that, while I was off the medication, there was a possibility my old cells could fight the new cells and therefore cause the SCD to return.

Naturally, I was apprehensive about this. The last thing I wanted was for me to face SCD in the manner of a pain crisis again. Mentally I refused to go back to that life. I also trusted my team of doctors and most importantly God. I believed that things would work out for the best. I knew I had to be fearless. I placed my trust in God and made preparations for surgery over the period of a few months. The day of surgery came and everything went well. I spent a few days at the facility and was eager to go home and recuperate. As I prepared to go home, I was given narcotics to help with the pain. Then it hit me. This was the first time in years I would be handling narcotics on my own. I struggled with the fear of getting addicted again. However, when I was home alone with these drugs, I realized I no longer had the desire to take it other than for pain. I realized that God had truly healed me of my addiction too. I realized as a child of God, I had to be accountable for my actions and that set me free from my bondage to this addiction. So the transformation I had gone through had rid me of the desire to abuse these narcotics. I was free!!! What a relief it was to know these drugs could no longer hold me hostage. Eventually I went back on the immunosuppressant as planned with no complications. God is good! It is almost a year post-surgery and I am doing very well. I am happy and grateful to God I sailed through this smoothly. I have returned to my normal long work schedule.

Sometimes, I wonder, what next. I am not sure what I am about to get hit with again in life. Like many people I wish I had a vision into my future but I do not. However, the one thing I know is that, I have decided I will no longer live in fear or worry. If He did it for me, He will do it again. I will continue to trust in Him. It has been a long journey. In fact, my life's journey thus far has been a long road with many twists and turns and many ups and downs. It has been a journey through mountains, hills, valleys, rain, snow, and one with many stops. I have been through and experienced a lot. On many days it felt as though there are more down turns than up. On other occasions, there are more mountains than plateaus. This journey although rough and turbulent, has made me who I am today. This course has made me stronger and more steadfast in faith. It has afforded me the opportunity to value life and value people. I could not have gone through this without the love, support and prayers of family and friends and even people I do not know. This road I've travelled has made me see first-hand the mighty hand of God. I have seen that nothing is impossible for Him. I mean nothing! Look at what He has brought me through? Look at what He has done for me. Know, my friend, that no matter what you are dealing with, you can call on Him and He will see you through it. He will answer in His own time according to His plan for you.

Chapter 25

I went through some tests, many of which I thought I would never overcome. There were occasions when I was so sick I thought and wished I would not see another day. The pain could be so excruciating; other complications would set in; and there were times when I begged silently that death would take me. But death did not take me as I had wished. Death did not claim me because God had a plan for me just like He does for you. I believe God healed me to show me He was the same God today as He was yesterday. I had completely stopped believing we serve a mighty God and one who hears our pleas. What was the point in continuing to believe when I had prayed for many years with no answer? Family, friends and even strangers had been praying for my healing for years, but, until the Transplant, I had not seen any change in my condition. In fact, my condition had seemed to be getting worse. Was Sickle Cell Disease not enough? Why the Osteomyelitis, the MS, the AVN, the Coma? At some point, I stopped believing in God, period! I had suffered way too long and prayed way too long and not seen a change in my situation. I had faith in God when it came to other things but definitely not when it came to my healing. Just like the man at the pool of Bethesda, I "sat" in my pain waiting for a change. Today, I know I just needed to exercise my faith by believing. No one could do it for me. It had to come from me.

Like the man at the Pool of Bethesda in John 5:1-14, I sat at the pool all those years waiting for an opportunity to jump in the pool when it was stirred so I could get my healing. All those years when the pool was stirred, I could not pick myself up to jump into it. All those years slipped by me because the time was not right. I sat at the pool wishing I could jump into it, wash myself and rid myself of these diseases. I did not have the strength or the courage to jump. I was broken in spirit and in faith. I was broken in more ways than I can describe. I had decided this was my fate. I watched others jump into the pool and got the help they needed. I watched other patients adapt so well to medications like Hydroxy Urea where the frequency of their pain crisis reduced. When the pool was stirred with Hydroxy Urea, I was unable to jump in to get the relief I desperately needed.

In hindsight, I realize it was not God's time for my healing yet. I sat and suffered for over thirty years at the Pool of Bethesda with many health conditions. Occasionally, I was envious of other patients who seemed to be doing so well. I was envious of other patients whose diseases were not manifesting as strongly or as painfully as mine were. When it came to Multiple Sclerosis, it was obvious my condition was not as bad as that of others. My journey with MS had not advanced further along like other patients. I met various patients suffering from MS and although I was happy my case was not as advanced as theirs, it was still very discouraging.

Seeing other MS patients whose condition was more advanced reminded of where I was heading. It was just a matter of time before I would lose mobility in different areas of my body. And that reminder was not easy to live with. Knowing what lay ahead for me, my future looked bleak.

At some point during my journey, I heard of some SCD patients in various parts of the country being cured through Bone Marrow Transplant. I was happy for them and wished I would get an opportunity like that. At the same time I thought an opportunity like this would never be presented to me due to my age and how advanced and complicated my case was. Most of the patients I had heard the success stories about only had one disease as far as I knew, and believed that contributed to their transplant being a success. In my case though, I was battling many conditions and complications. In my mind this complicated my case for a possible bone marrow transplant. I had rationalized the reason why I would not be a candidate for this procedure. Little did I know Jesus was walking towards the pool of Bethesda and at the appointed time, would offer me a hand to receive the healing I had hoped for. It all had to be in His time and not mine. Everything He does is ultimately for His glory. It had to be in His time and not mine. He had a plan for me. He met me where I was in life and used my mother's bone marrow to heal me. I believe God waited this long, over thirty seven years to seize this opportunity to prove me wrong. And HE did! He proved me so wrong my faith and that of others have been renewed and strengthened. Nowadays when I face challenges whether it is health related or not, I may get anxious for a little while, but in remembering my moments of hope, my faith calms me down. I quickly gather myself, and remember what God has done knowing that it will all work out for my good in the end. I know the God I serve and nothing can change my mind.

I wake up occasionally wondering if this is really me. Yes I do! My life is completely different from what it used to be and it amazes me. When I say my life has made a 360 degree turn, I mean it really has. I was always in pain and miserable. I was unhappy and depressed. I was angry and frustrated with God and at my life. One of the nurses that had cared for me at NIH over the years once said to me, "Jennifer, I could tell the pain you were going through weighed heavily on you that it affected every area of your life." Yes, she was right; the pain consumed my life and everything I did. Depression clouded my vision in life. There was no genuine joy in my heart and soul. Though I was physically present, emotionally, I was not there. I was on so many medications for relief. I sought not only relief but also an escape with these medications. Relying on these medications gave me a reason not to engage or get involved with anything.

Since being cured of Multiple Sclerosis and Sickle Cell Disease, my life has improved dramatically. I am a completely different person compared to who I was before. I am more engaging, more humorous and more outgoing. I enjoy engaging in many different activities including interacting with my nephews and nieces who are all in their pre-teenage years. I complain less and see a positive side in every situation. I am less angry and a joy to be around. I have become more helpful and supportive. I am no longer self-centered, uncaring and inconsiderate of other people's feelings.

God has given me a second chance at life and I am living it. I refuse to be the person I used to be. By His grace and mercy, I have evolved and continue to evolve daily. I am a better person. I prayed for years for God to reveal what my purpose is in this life. I realized my purpose is to share my story to encourage others who may be experiencing a myriad of health issues. And also to let others know God is the same God He used to be in ancient days. So we need to trust Him and ask for a strong faith to serve Him.

Conclusion

To answer the questions I raised in the introduction, my dear friend, know that God is real. Know that God is good. In life we will go through struggles; we will go through challenges. Through it all God is with us if we call on Him. Some days it may seem as though we are ready to give up; ready not to fight anymore. In fact, some days we may wish life would end so the pain, frustration, depression and darkness will also end. But know that if your work here on earth is not finished, you are not going anywhere. When you wake up to another day, know things will get better; know that things will change. It may be tough facing another day; it may be tough facing another health challenge; it may be tough getting out of bed and making it to another doctor's appointment; and it may be difficult putting a smile on your face. In all this remember to put your faith and trust in him. Continue to trust in God and immerse yourself in praise and prayer and the love and support from friends and family will see you through it all. Know God is in your corner no matter what. It may not seem like it, but He is. Trust Him and call on Him at all times. Trust in Him to take you through this journey and come out with victory.

He is our source of hope and victory. We are nothing without Him. I recall many nights when I was in so much pain I could barely move. There were nights I thought and wished would be my last. Yes, the pain was too much to bear, too much to want to face another hour, let alone another day. Through it all I would call on Him even though I did not have a strong faith then. Yet, He brought me through those difficult times because He had other plans for me. He held my hand and assisted me in traversing some of my life's toughest times. He helped me in plowing through and overcoming these mountains I faced. Yes, I call them mountains. For example, a period in time I considered a mountain was while in a coma as a result of complications from medications for MS that interfered with the SCD. All those antibodies I had developed as a result of numerous blood transfusions that will forever be a part of me, was also a mountain and there were more.

    I look back on what my life was like and I cannot fathom I went through all that and I am still here. I believe there is a reason for me to still be here. I know there is a purpose for me to fulfill and writing this memoir is a part of it. I refuse to dwell on how difficult it was. Rather I choose to reflect on it and use it as an impetus, to inform others and also remind myself how great God is. He still works miracles. Remember He is the same yesterday and today. He has done it for me and will do it again. He can do it for you, trust in Him. These eyes have shed many tears and I still do sometimes. The tears were for pain and frustration. Today, they are tears of joy. I am still amazed at the transformation I see in my life daily. The tears I shed come from a place of joy and contentment with my health. Although I still have some challenges ahead of me, I know my faith in God will pull me through anything.

After everything I have been through, I know I will be alright, come what may. I have gained strength and confidence I have never had before. I am transformed but still a work in progress.

As I conclude this memoir, on the 25th day of January, 2018, I do not know what my future holds. I have been advised by my medical team at the NIH my chimerism levels are low, and if they should fall any lower than where they are at 18%, I will have to get re-transplanted. Chimerism is the state in which donor cells have engrafted in the recipient. As a result, a full donor chimerism implies that 100% of bone marrow and blood cells are of donor origin. With this news, I may have to go through a second transplant. At this point in life I have decided not to worry or get anxious about anything. Again, I am trusting in and relying on God, because He knows best. He knows the plans He has for me. If I have to go through a second transplant, I know God will give me the strength and courage to do that. Come what may, I will come out on top with God on my side. Although it is certainly not my wish to undergo this procedure again, I know it will all work out for my good.

Sharing my experiences in this book is not an attempt to seek pity or draw attention to myself. Rather, this book is to share my story with the hopes of encouraging others. I hope to let people know we all face challenges in life. Trials come in various forms as we tread through this journey called life. Though some trials are tougher than others, they all come to strengthen us in faith and character. Stem cell has changed my life in many ways. This procedure, has now allowed me to live life free of SCD and MS. The pain crisis has been eliminated. The pain that consumed my life daily and the long list of medications have been taken away. Not having to deal with all of that is what has caused a transformation. But before the transformation, I had to get to a place of trust and surrender so God could do His work. I had to get to that place so God's hand could move in my life and grant me the healing I had prayed for, for so many years. In surrendering and trusting Him, I allowed God to take control and work out His miracle in my life.

This miracle has brought with it great transformation. I would never have dreamt to be in the space I am in at this moment. I have complete and total trust in Him. I am courageous and outspoken about a lot of things, most especially my healing. I am not the shy timid person I used to be. I would never even have dreamt of writing this memoir, had I not gone through this journey. I am doing things I never dreamt I would. I am more confident and my faith is stronger than it has ever been. God is good!

My friend, I urge you to stay encouraged and to have trust in Him for He will do it in His own time and for His glory. Stay blessed!

"For no word from God will ever fail."
(New International Version, Luke 1:37)

Works Cited

"Accra, Ghana (Ca. 1500-) | The Black Past: Remembered and Reclaimed." St. Clair, Stephanie (1886–1969) | The Black Past: Remembered and Reclaimed, www.blackpast.org/gah/accra-ghana-ca-1500.

"African Crafts Market." Zulu Tribe, www.africancraftsmarket.com/african-tribes/ashanti-people.html.

"Bone Marrow Transplant Glossary." UCSF Benioff Children's Hospital - San Francisco, www.ucsfbenioffchildrens.org/education/bone_marrow_transplant_glossary/.

"Brain Aneurysm Basics." Brain Aneurysm Foundation, www.bafound.org/about-brain-aneurysms/brain-aneurysm-basics/.

Bridges, Kenneth R. "Stroke in Sickle Cell Disease." A Brief History of Sickle Cell Disease, sickle.bwh.harvard.edu/stroke.html.

"Elmina Castle." Wikipedia, Wikimedia Foundation, 27 July 2018, en.wikipedia.org/wiki/Elmina_Castle.

Hill, Bryan. "Elmina Castle and Its Dark History of Enslavement, Torture, and Death." Ancient Origins, Ancient Origins, www.ancient-origins.net/ancient-places-africa/elmina-castle-and-its-dark-history-enslavement-torture-and-death-003450.

"Korle Bu Teaching Hospital." About Us - Korle Bu Teaching Hospital, www.kbth.gov.gh/2/about-us.html.

"Malaria: Causes, Symptoms, and Diagnosis." Healthline,

Healthline Media, www.healthline.com/health/malaria.

New International Version, Acts 3:6. Zondervan, 2011.

New International Version, John 5:1-14. Zondervan, 2011.

New International Version, Luke 1:37. Zondervan, 2011.

"Osteomyelitis." WebMD, WebMD, www.webmd.com/diabetes/osteomyeltis-treatment-diagnosis-symptoms.

"Sickle Cell Disease." KidsHealth, The Nemours Foundation, July 2018,kidshealth.org/ChildrensHospitalPittsburgh/en/teens/sickle-cell-anemia.html.

"Sickle Cell Disease." National Heart Lung and Blood Institute, U.S. Department of Health and Human Services, www.nhlbi.nih.gov/health-topics/sickle-cell-disease.

"Stem Cell Transplantation for Cancer Treatment | CTCA." CancerCenter.com, 1 Jan. 1AD, www.cancercenter.com/treatments/stem-cell-transplantation/?source=GGLPS01.

UpToDate, www.uptodate.com/contents/bone-and-joint-complications-in-sickle-cell-disease.

ViewAdmin. "History of the Central Region Ghana and the Infamous Cape Coast." ViewGhana Things to Do in Ghana from Festivals, Events Music, 16 Feb. 2018, viewghana.com/history-of-central-region-ghana-infamous-cape-coast/.

Contact Information and Bulk Ordering

E-mail & Bulk Ordering
jenn.nsenkyire@gmail.com

Website
www.jennifernsenkyire.com

Facebook
jennifer.nsenkyire.5

Twitter
JNsenkyire

Instagram
mypoolofbethesda